AFIB DIET

COOKBOOK

DR. MAUREEN MOORE

TABLE OF CONTENT

CHAPTER ONE

Introduction

Using an atrial fibrillation (AFib) diet cookbook can be a helpful and practical way to manage your diet and support heart health. Here are some general steps on how to use an AFib diet cookbook effectively:

Understand the AFib Diet Guidelines: Familiarize yourself with the dietary recommendations for managing AFib. These guidelines often include reducing sodium intake, maintaining a healthy weight, limiting caffeine and alcohol, and emphasizing nutrient-dense foods.

Choose a Cookbook with AFib-Friendly Recipes: Select a cookbook specifically tailored for individuals with AFib or heart health concerns. Look for cookbooks authored by nutritionists, cardiologists, or experts in the field of heart health.

Read the Introduction and Guidelines: Begin by reading the introduction and guidelines provided in the cookbook. This section often includes information about the principles of the

AFib diet, essential nutrients, and tips for creating balanced meals.

Meal Planning: Plan your meals based on the recipes provided in the cookbook. Consider incorporating a variety of fruits, vegetables, lean proteins, whole grains, and heart-healthy fats. Aim for balanced and portion-controlled meals.

Grocery Shopping: Create a shopping list based on the ingredients required for the recipes you've selected. Focus on fresh, whole foods and try to minimize processed or high-sodium items.

Cooking and Preparation: Follow the recipes step by step. Pay attention to cooking techniques and portion sizes. Cooking at home allows you to have better control over the ingredients and preparation methods.

Experiment with Flavors: Don't be afraid to experiment with herbs and spices to add flavor to your dishes without relying on excessive salt. Many AFib diet cookbooks provide suggestions for flavorful, heart-healthy seasonings.

Monitor Sodium Intake: Keep track of your sodium intake, as excessive salt can contribute to fluid retention and affect heart health. The cookbook may provide guidance on how to season dishes without relying on salt.

Stay Hydrated: Adequate hydration is crucial for heart health. Ensure you are drinking enough water throughout the day, and consider incorporating hydrating foods like fruits and vegetables into your meals.

Listen to Your Body:Pay attention to how your body responds to different foods. If you notice any adverse reactions or if certain ingredients exacerbate your AFib symptoms, consult with your healthcare provider.

Consult with Healthcare Professionals: Before making significant changes to your diet, especially if you have pre-existing health conditions like AFib, it's essential to consult with your healthcare team. They can provide personalized advice based on your specific health needs.

Remember, an AFib diet cookbook is a tool to guide you toward healthier eating habits, but individual dietary needs may vary. Always seek guidance from healthcare professionals for personalized advice based on your health condition and history.

Understanding Afib Diet Cookbook

Understanding and effectively using an atrial fibrillation (AFib) diet cookbook involves several key steps. Here's a guide to help you navigate and make the most of such a resource:

Read the Introduction: Start by reading the introduction section of the cookbook. This often provides valuable information about the principles of the AFib diet, the importance of specific nutrients, and general guidelines for managing AFib through nutrition.

Familiarize Yourself with AFib-Friendly Foods: Understand the types of foods that are typically recommended for individuals with AFib. These often include fruits, vegetables, whole grains, lean proteins, and heart-healthy fats.

Learn about Restrictive or Limiting Factors: Identify any foods or ingredients that the cookbook suggests limiting or avoiding. Common restrictions may include sodium, caffeine, alcohol, and processed foods. Understanding these limitations is crucial for following the AFib diet.

Take Note of Portion Sizes: Pay attention to recommended portion sizes for various foods. Portion control is an essential aspect of managing AFib, as overeating can contribute to weight gain and other cardiovascular issues.

Explore Sample Meal Plans: Many AFib diet cookbooks provide sample meal plans or suggestions. Study these plans to see how a balanced and AFib-friendly day of eating is structured. This can help you plan your meals and snacks.

Understand Seasoning Alternatives: Given that excessive salt is often restricted in an AFib diet, learn about alternative ways to season your food. The cookbook may suggest herbs, spices, and other flavor enhancers that can add taste without increasing sodium intake.

Adapt Recipes to Your Preferences: While following the cookbook's recipes, feel free to adapt them based on your taste preferences. Experiment with different herbs, spices, and cooking techniques to make the meals enjoyable for you.

Create a Grocery List: Use the recipes provided to create a comprehensive grocery list. Ensure you have all the necessary ingredients, and focus on purchasing fresh, whole foods.

Cook Mindfully: When preparing meals, follow the recipes carefully. Pay attention to cooking methods, suggested cooking times, and any specific instructions related to preserving nutritional value.

Stay Hydrated: Understand the importance of hydration in managing AFib. Many AFib diet plans encourage adequate water intake. Consider incorporating hydrating foods like fruits and vegetables into your meals.

Monitor and Assess: Keep a record of your dietary choices and how your body responds. Monitor any changes in symptoms or overall well-being. This information can be valuable when discussing your diet with healthcare professionals.

Seek Professional Guidance: Before making significant changes to your diet, consult with your healthcare provider or a registered dietitian. They can provide personalized advice based on your specific health condition, medical history, and dietary needs.

Remember that an AFib diet cookbook is a tool to guide you toward healthier eating, but individual responses to foods can vary. Always consult with healthcare professionals for personalized advice and ensure that any dietary changes align with your overall health goals.

Principles of afib diet cookbook

The principles of an atrial fibrillation (AFib) diet cookbook are centered around promoting heart health and managing the symptoms associated with AFib. Here are some common principles often found in an AFib diet cookbook:

Reducing Sodium Intake: High sodium levels can contribute to fluid retention and high blood pressure, exacerbating AFib symptoms. The cookbook typically emphasizes the importance of reducing sodium intake by choosing fresh, whole foods and minimizing processed and salty foods.

Balanced Nutrition: The cookbook encourages a balanced intake of macronutrients (carbohydrates, proteins, and fats) and micronutrients (vitamins and minerals). This helps maintain overall health and supports heart function.

Limiting Caffeine and Stimulants: Caffeine and other stimulants can potentially trigger or worsen AFib symptoms. The cookbook may recommend limiting or avoiding caffeinated beverages and other stimulants.

Moderating Alcohol Consumption: Excessive alcohol intake can contribute to heart issues. The cookbook typically advises moderation in alcohol consumption or, in some cases, complete avoidance.

Emphasizing Heart-Healthy Fats: The focus is on incorporating heart-healthy fats, such as those found in avocados, nuts, seeds, and olive oil, while limiting saturated and trans fats.

Lean protein sources, such as poultry, fish, beans, and legumes, are often recommended over high-fat or processed meat options.

Incorporating Whole Grains: Whole grains provide fiber and essential nutrients. The cookbook may encourage the consumption of whole grains like brown rice, quinoa, oats, and whole wheat.

Including Nutrient-Dense Foods: Nutrient-dense foods, such as fruits and vegetables, are rich in vitamins, minerals, and antioxidants. The cookbook likely features recipes incorporating a variety of colorful fruits and vegetables.

Managing Portion Sizes: Portion control is crucial for weight management and overall heart health. The cookbook may provide guidance on appropriate portion sizes to prevent overeating.

Hydration: Staying adequately hydrated is essential for heart health. The cookbook may recommend water as the primary beverage and suggest hydrating foods like water-rich fruits and vegetables.

Monitoring and Listening to Your Body: The cookbook often encourages individuals to pay attention to their bodies, noting how specific foods or meals may impact AFib symptoms. It emphasizes self-awareness and encourages adjusting the diet based on individual responses.

Adaptable Recipes: The cookbook likely features adaptable recipes that accommodate dietary preferences, restrictions, or allergies. This flexibility ensures that individuals can enjoy flavorful meals while adhering to AFib diet principles.

Regular Physical Activity: While not directly related to diet, many AFib diet cookbooks may stress the importance of regular physical activity as part of an overall heart-healthy lifestyle.

Stress Management: Chronic stress can contribute to AFib symptoms. The cookbook may offer tips on stress management techniques to complement dietary changes.

It's important to note that individual dietary needs can vary, and these principles may be adapted based on specific health conditions and personal preferences. Always consult with healthcare professionals or a registered dietitian before making significant changes to your diet, especially if you have AFib or other health concerns.

Benefits of Afib Diet

Adopting an atrial fibrillation (AFib) diet can offer several benefits for individuals managing this heart condition. While individual responses may vary, the following are potential benefits associated with an AFib-friendly diet:

Heart Health Support: An AFib diet is designed to support overall heart health by emphasizing nutrient-dense foods that contribute to cardiovascular well-being. This includes fruits, vegetables, whole grains, lean proteins, and heart-healthy fats.

Blood Pressure Management: By reducing sodium intake and focusing on foods that promote blood vessel health, an AFib diet may help manage blood pressure. Controlling blood pressure is crucial for individuals with AFib, as high blood pressure can contribute to heart rhythm issues.

Weight Management: The emphasis on balanced nutrition and portion control in an AFib diet can contribute to weight management. Maintaining a healthy weight is important for overall cardiovascular health and may help alleviate symptoms of AFib.

Reduced Risk of Stroke: AFib is associated with an increased risk of stroke. Following an AFib diet that includes foods with anti-inflammatory and antioxidant properties may contribute to a lower risk of stroke.

Balanced Blood Sugar Levels: Choosing whole grains and nutrient-dense carbohydrates as part of an AFib diet can help regulate blood sugar levels. This is particularly important for individuals with diabetes, as diabetes is a common coexisting condition with AFib.

Anti-Inflammatory Effects: Certain foods included in an AFib diet, such as fatty fish, nuts, and berries, have anti-inflammatory properties. Chronic inflammation is linked to various cardiovascular issues, and an anti-inflammatory diet may help manage inflammation.

Improved Lipid Profile: Consuming heart-healthy fats, such as those found in avocados, olive oil, and fatty fish, can positively impact lipid profiles by raising high-density lipoprotein (HDL) cholesterol and lowering low-density lipoprotein (LDL) cholesterol.

Symptom Management: Some individuals with AFib may experience symptoms such as palpitations or fatigue. An AFib diet that minimizes triggers, such as caffeine and alcohol, and promotes stable blood sugar levels may contribute to symptom management.

Enhanced Nutrient Intake: The emphasis on a variety of fruits and vegetables in an AFib diet ensures a diverse intake of essential vitamins, minerals, and antioxidants, supporting overall health.

Better Hydration: An AFib diet often encourages adequate water intake. Staying well-hydrated is essential for cardiovascular health, as dehydration can contribute to irregular heart rhythms.

Increased Awareness of Dietary Choices: Adopting an AFib diet promotes greater awareness of dietary choices and their impact on heart health. This increased awareness can empower individuals to make informed decisions about their nutrition.

It's important to note that while an AFib diet can offer these potential benefits, it is just one component of a comprehensive approach to managing AFib. Individuals with AFib should work closely with healthcare professionals, including cardiologists and dietitians, to tailor dietary recommendations to their specific health needs and overall treatment plan.

Tips on Afib Diet

Managing atrial fibrillation (AFib) through diet involves making heart-healthy choices to support overall cardiovascular health and potentially alleviate symptoms. Here are some tips for an AFib-friendly diet:

Limit Sodium Intake: Reduce the consumption of high-sodium foods, as excessive salt can contribute to fluid retention and increase blood pressure. Choose fresh, whole foods and minimize processed and packaged items.

Choose Nutrient-Dense Foods: Emphasize a variety of nutrient-dense foods, including fruits, vegetables, whole grains, lean proteins, and heart-healthy fats. These foods provide essential vitamins, minerals, and antioxidants.

Control Portion Sizes: Practice portion control to manage calorie intake and support weight management. Overeating can strain the cardiovascular system and exacerbate AFib symptoms.

Moderate Caffeine Intake: Limit or moderate caffeine consumption, as excessive caffeine can trigger or worsen AFib symptoms in some individuals. Be mindful of coffee, tea, energy drinks, and certain medications containing caffeine.

Limit Alcohol Consumption: Moderation is key when it comes to alcohol. Limit alcohol intake, as excessive alcohol consumption can contribute to AFib. Consult with your healthcare provider to determine a safe level of alcohol consumption for your individual health.

Include Omega-3 Fatty Acids: Incorporate sources of omega-3 fatty acids, such as fatty fish (salmon, mackerel, sardines), flaxseeds, chia seeds, and walnuts. Omega-3s have anti-inflammatory properties that may benefit heart health.

Choose Lean Proteins: Opt for lean protein sources like poultry, fish, beans, legumes, and tofu. Limit intake of high-fat or processed meats, as they can contribute to cardiovascular issues.

Hydrate Adequately: Stay well-hydrated by drinking water throughout the day. Dehydration can contribute to irregular heart rhythms, so maintaining proper hydration is crucial.

Limit Refined Sugars: Minimize the intake of foods and beverages high in refined sugars. Focus on natural sources of sweetness, such as fruits, and be mindful of added sugars in processed foods.

Incorporate Fiber-Rich Foods: Choose fiber-rich foods like whole grains, fruits, vegetables, and legumes. Fiber supports digestive health and may have positive effects on heart health.

Monitor Potassium Intake: Include potassium-rich foods in your diet, such as bananas, oranges, spinach, sweet potatoes, and tomatoes. Potassium is essential for maintaining a healthy heart rhythm.

Be Mindful of Trigger Foods: Identify and be mindful of foods that may act as triggers for AFib symptoms. Common triggers include caffeine, alcohol, spicy foods, and certain food additives.

Cook with Heart-Healthy Oils: Use heart-healthy oils like olive oil or canola oil for cooking. These oils contain monounsaturated fats that support cardiovascular health.

Consider Meal Timing: Pay attention to meal timing, as some individuals may experience symptoms after consuming large meals. Eating smaller, more frequent meals throughout the day may be beneficial.

Work with a Healthcare Professional: Consult with your healthcare provider or a registered dietitian to create a personalized AFib diet plan tailored to your specific health needs, medications, and lifestyle.

Remember, individual responses to dietary changes can vary, and it's crucial to work with healthcare professionals to determine the most suitable dietary approach for your unique health condition and needs.

Following a well-structured atrial fibrillation (AFib) diet involves adhering to specific guidelines that aim to support heart health and manage symptoms associated with AFib. Here are general guidelines for an AFib-friendly diet:

Reduce Sodium Intake: Limit the consumption of high-sodium foods, as excess salt can contribute to fluid retention and elevate blood pressure. Choose fresh, whole foods and be mindful of sodium content in processed items.

Choose Nutrient-Dense Foods: Prioritize nutrient-dense foods, including fruits, vegetables, whole grains, lean proteins, and heart-healthy fats. These foods provide essential vitamins, minerals, and antioxidants.

Control Portion Sizes: Practice portion control to manage caloric intake and support weight management. Maintaining a healthy weight is crucial for overall cardiovascular health.

Moderate Caffeine Intake: Limit caffeine consumption, as excessive caffeine can potentially trigger AFib episodes in some individuals. Monitor your sensitivity to caffeine and adjust your intake accordingly.

Limit Alcohol Consumption: Moderation is key when it comes to alcohol. Limit alcohol intake, as excessive consumption can contribute to AFib. Consult with your healthcare provider to determine a safe level of alcohol consumption for your individual health.

Include Omega-3 Fatty Acids: Incorporate sources of omega-3 fatty acids, such as fatty fish (salmon, mackerel, sardines), flaxseeds, chia seeds, and walnuts. Omega-3s have anti-inflammatory properties that may benefit heart health.

Choose Lean Proteins: Opt for lean protein sources like poultry, fish, beans, legumes, and tofu. Limit the intake of high-fat or processed meats to reduce the risk of cardiovascular issues.

Hydrate Adequately: Stay well-hydrated by drinking water throughout the day. Dehydration can contribute to irregular heart rhythms, so maintaining proper hydration is important.

Limit Refined Sugars: Minimize the consumption of foods and beverages high in refined sugars. Focus on natural sources of sweetness, such as fruits, and be mindful of added sugars in processed foods.

Incorporate Fiber-Rich Foods: Choose fiber-rich foods like whole grains, fruits, vegetables, and legumes. Fiber supports digestive health and may have positive effects on heart health.

Monitor Potassium Intake: Include potassium-rich foods in your diet, such as bananas, oranges, spinach, sweet potatoes, and tomatoes. Potassium is crucial for maintaining a healthy heart rhythm.

Be Mindful of Trigger Foods: Identify and be mindful of foods that may act as triggers for AFib symptoms. Common triggers include caffeine, alcohol, spicy foods, and certain food additives.

Cook with Heart-Healthy Oils: Use heart-healthy oils like olive oil or canola oil for cooking. These oils contain monounsaturated fats that support cardiovascular health.

Consider Meal Timing: Pay attention to meal timing, as some individuals may experience symptoms after consuming large meals. Eating smaller, more frequent meals throughout the day may be beneficial.

Work with Healthcare Professionals: Collaborate with your healthcare provider or a registered dietitian to create a personalized AFib diet plan based on your specific health condition, medications, and lifestyle.

These guidelines provide a foundation for an AFib-friendly diet, but it's essential to tailor dietary choices based on individual health needs and consult with healthcare professionals for personalized advice.

CHAPTER TWO

RECIPES FOR AFIB DIET COOKBOOK

1. Salmon and Quinoa Stuffed Bell Peppers

Ingredients:

2 bell peppers, halved

1 cup cooked quinoa

1 can (6 oz) salmon, drained and flaked

1 cup cherry tomatoes, halved

1/4 cup feta cheese, crumbled

2 tablespoons fresh parsley, chopped

Salt and pepper to taste

Instructions:

Preheat the oven to 375°F (190°C).

In a bowl, combine cooked quinoa, flaked salmon, cherry tomatoes, feta cheese, and fresh parsley. Season with salt and pepper.

Stuff each bell pepper half with the mixture.

Place the stuffed peppers on a baking sheet and bake for 20-25 minutes or until peppers are tender.

Health Benefits:

Salmon provides omega-3 fatty acids, which support heart health.

Quinoa is a whole grain rich in fiber and essential nutrients.

Bell peppers offer vitamins and antioxidants.

Cooking Time: Approximately 25 minutes

2. Mediterranean Chickpea Salad

Ingredients:

1 can (15 oz) chickpeas, drained and rinsed

1 cucumber, diced

1 cup cherry tomatoes, halved

1/2 red onion, finely chopped

1/4 cup Kalamata olives, sliced

1/4 cup feta cheese, crumbled

2 tablespoons extra-virgin olive oil

1 tablespoon red wine vinegar

Fresh oregano, chopped (optional)

Salt and pepper to taste

Instructions:

In a large bowl, combine chickpeas, cucumber, cherry tomatoes, red onion, olives, and feta cheese.

In a small bowl, whisk together olive oil, red wine vinegar, and fresh oregano.

Pour the dressing over the salad and toss gently. Season with salt and pepper.

Chill in the refrigerator for at least 30 minutes before serving.

Health Benefits:

Chickpeas provide fiber and plant-based protein.

Olive oil is rich in monounsaturated fats, beneficial for heart health.

Fresh vegetables offer vitamins and antioxidants.

Cooking Time: Approximately 15 minutes

3. Baked Sweet Potato and Kale Hash

Ingredients:

2 medium sweet potatoes, peeled and diced

2 cups kale, chopped

1 red bell pepper, diced

1 onion, finely chopped

2 cloves garlic, minced

2 tablespoons olive oil

1 teaspoon smoked paprika

Salt and pepper to taste

Instructions:

Preheat the oven to 400°F (200°C).

In a large bowl, toss sweet potatoes, kale, red bell pepper, onion, and garlic with olive oil and smoked paprika.

Spread the mixture on a baking sheet in a single layer.

Bake for 25-30 minutes or until sweet potatoes are tender, stirring halfway through.

Health Benefits:

Sweet potatoes are rich in fiber, vitamins, and antioxidants.

Kale provides essential nutrients, including vitamin K and folate.

Olive oil contains heart-healthy monounsaturated fats.

Cooking Time: Approximately 30 minutes

4. Chicken and Vegetable Skewers

Ingredients:

1 pound boneless, skinless chicken breasts, cut into cubes

Bell peppers (assorted colors), onions, and cherry tomatoes for skewering

2 tablespoons olive oil

1 teaspoon dried oregano

1 teaspoon garlic powder

Salt and pepper to taste

Instructions:

Preheat the grill or grill pan.

In a bowl, mix chicken cubes with olive oil, oregano, garlic powder, salt, and pepper.

Thread chicken and vegetables onto skewers.

Grill for 10-12 minutes, turning occasionally, until chicken is cooked through.

Health Benefits:

Chicken is a lean protein source.

Bell peppers provide vitamins and antioxidants.

Cooking Time: Approximately 12 minutes

5. Quinoa Salad with Avocado and Black Beans

Ingredients:

1 cup cooked quinoa

1 can (15 oz) black beans, drained and rinsed

1 avocado, diced

1 cup corn kernels (fresh or frozen)

1/4 cup cilantro, chopped

Juice of 1 lime

2 tablespoons olive oil

Salt and cumin to taste

Instructions:

In a large bowl, combine quinoa, black beans, diced avocado, corn, and cilantro.

In a small bowl, whisk together lime juice, olive oil, salt, and cumin.

Pour the dressing over the salad and toss gently.

Serve chilled.

Health Benefits:

Quinoa provides fiber and essential nutrients.

Avocado offers healthy fats and potassium.

Cooking Time: Approximately 15 minutes

6. Salmon and Vegetable Foil Packets

Ingredients:

2 salmon fillets

1 zucchini, sliced

1 yellow squash, sliced

Cherry tomatoes

2 tablespoons olive oil

Lemon slices

Fresh dill, chopped

Salt and pepper to taste

Instructions:

Preheat the oven to 375°F (190°C).

Place each salmon fillet on a piece of aluminum foil.

Surround each fillet with zucchini, yellow squash, and cherry tomatoes.

Drizzle olive oil over the salmon and vegetables. Season with salt and pepper.

Seal the foil packets and bake for 15-20 minutes or until salmon is cooked through.

Health Benefits:

Salmon is rich in omega-3 fatty acids.

Zucchini and yellow squash provide vitamins and fiber.

Cooking Time: Approximately 20 minutes

7. Spinach and Feta Stuffed Chicken Breast

Ingredients:

2 boneless, skinless chicken breasts

2 cups fresh spinach, chopped

1/4 cup feta cheese, crumbled

1 clove garlic, minced

1 tablespoon olive oil

Salt and pepper to taste

Instructions:

Preheat the oven to 375°F (190°C).

In a skillet, sauté spinach and garlic in olive oil until wilted.

Butterfly each chicken breast and stuff with sautéed spinach and feta.

Season with salt and pepper.

Bake for 25-30 minutes or until chicken is cooked through.

Health Benefits:

Spinach is a nutrient-dense leafy green.

Feta cheese adds a flavorful touch with moderate fat content.

Cooking Time: Approximately 30 minutes

8. Vegetable and Lentil Soup

Ingredients:

1 cup dried green or brown lentils, rinsed

1 onion, chopped

2 carrots, diced

2 celery stalks, chopped

3 cloves garlic, minced

1 can (14 oz) diced tomatoes

4 cups low-sodium vegetable broth

1 teaspoon cumin

1 teaspoon paprika

Salt and pepper to taste

Instructions:

In a large pot, combine lentils, onion, carrots, celery, garlic, diced tomatoes, and vegetable broth.

Season with cumin, paprika, salt, and pepper.

Bring to a boil, then reduce heat and simmer for 25-30 minutes or until lentils are tender.

Health Benefits:

Lentils are a good source of plant-based protein and fiber.

Vegetables provide essential vitamins and minerals.

Cooking Time: Approximately 30 minutes

9. Turkey and Quinoa Stuffed Peppers

Ingredients:

4 bell peppers, halved

1 pound ground turkey

1 cup cooked quinoa

1 can (14 oz) diced tomatoes, drained

1 cup black beans, drained and rinsed

1 teaspoon cumin

1 teaspoon chili powder

Salt and pepper to taste

Shredded cheese (optional for topping)

Instructions:

Preheat the oven to 375°F (190°C).

In a skillet, cook ground turkey until browned. Drain excess fat.

In a bowl, mix cooked turkey, quinoa, diced tomatoes, black beans, cumin, chili powder, salt, and pepper.

Stuff each bell pepper half with the mixture.

Bake for 25-30 minutes. Top with shredded cheese if desired and bake for an additional 5 minutes.

Health Benefits:

Ground turkey

10. Shrimp and Broccoli Stir-Fry

Ingredients:

1-pound shrimp, peeled and deveined

2 cups broccoli florets

1 red bell pepper, sliced

2 cloves garlic, minced

2 tablespoons low-sodium soy sauce

1 tablespoon honey

1 tablespoon sesame oil

1 teaspoon ginger, grated

Brown rice for serving

Instructions:

In a wok or skillet, heat sesame oil over medium-high heat.

Add shrimp and stir-fry until pink. Remove from the wok.

In the same wok, stir-fry broccoli, bell pepper, and garlic until vegetables are crisp-tender.

Return shrimp to the wok, add soy sauce, honey, and grated ginger. Toss until well-coated.

Serve over brown rice.

Health Benefits:

Shrimp provides lean protein.

Broccoli is rich in vitamins and antioxidants.

Cooking Time: Approximately 15 minutes

11. Mango and Avocado Salad with Grilled Chicken

Ingredients:

2 boneless, skinless chicken breasts

1 mango, diced

1 avocado, diced

1 cup cherry tomatoes, halved

1/4 cup red onion, finely chopped

2 tablespoons fresh cilantro, chopped

Juice of 1 lime

1 tablespoon olive oil

Salt and pepper to taste

Instructions:

Season chicken breasts with salt and pepper, then grill until fully cooked.

Slice grilled chicken into strips.

In a large bowl, combine mango, avocado, cherry tomatoes, red onion, and cilantro.

Toss with lime juice and olive oil.

Top the salad with grilled chicken strips.

Health Benefits:

Mango and avocado provide vitamins and healthy fats.

Grilled chicken offers lean protein.

Cooking Time: Approximately 20 minutes

12. Lemon Garlic Roasted Vegetables

Ingredients:

Assorted vegetables (zucchini, carrots, cherry tomatoes, Brussels sprouts)

2 tablespoons olive oil

2 cloves garlic, minced

Zest of 1 lemon

1 tablespoon fresh thyme leaves

Salt and pepper to taste

Instructions:

Preheat the oven to 400°F (200°C).

Cut vegetables into bite-sized pieces.

In a bowl, toss vegetables with olive oil, minced garlic, lemon zest, thyme, salt, and pepper.

Spread vegetables on a baking sheet in a single layer.

Roast for 20-25 minutes or until vegetables are golden brown.

Health Benefits:

Assorted vegetables provide a variety of nutrients.

Olive oil contains heart-healthy monounsaturated fats.

Cooking Time: Approximately 25 minutes

13. Tuna and White Bean Salad

Ingredients:

2 cans (5 oz each) tuna, drained

1 can (15 oz) white beans, drained and rinsed

1 cucumber, diced

1 red onion, finely chopped

1/4 cup parsley, chopped

Juice of 1 lemon

2 tablespoons olive oil

Salt and pepper to taste

Instructions:

In a large bowl, combine tuna, white beans, cucumber, red onion, and parsley.

Whisk together lemon juice, olive oil, salt, and pepper.

Pour the dressing over the salad and toss gently.

Health Benefits:

Tuna provides protein and omega-3 fatty acids.

White beans offer fiber and essential nutrients.

Cooking Time: Approximately 10 minutes

14. Stuffed Portobello Mushrooms with Quinoa and Spinach

Ingredients:

4 large Portobello mushrooms

1 cup cooked quinoa

2 cups fresh spinach, chopped

1/4 cup sun-dried tomatoes, chopped

1/4 cup feta cheese, crumbled

2 tablespoons balsamic vinegar

1 tablespoon olive oil

Salt and pepper to taste

Instructions:

Preheat the oven to 375°F (190°C).

Remove the stems from Portobello mushrooms and brush with olive oil.

In a bowl, mix cooked quinoa, chopped spinach, sun-dried tomatoes, and feta.

Stuff each mushroom cap with the quinoa mixture.

Drizzle balsamic vinegar over the top.

Bake for 20-25 minutes or until mushrooms are tender.

Health Benefits:

Portobello mushrooms provide a meaty texture.

Quinoa and spinach offer nutrients and fiber.

Cooking Time: Approximately 25 minutes

15. Cauliflower and Chickpea Curry

Ingredients:

1 cauliflower, cut into florets

1 can (15 oz) chickpeas, drained and rinsed

1 onion, finely chopped

2 cloves garlic, minced

1 can (14 oz) diced tomatoes

1 can (14 oz) coconut milk

2 tablespoons curry powder

1 teaspoon turmeric

Salt and pepper to taste

Fresh cilantro for garnish

Instructions:

In a large pot, sauté onions and garlic until softened.

Add cauliflower, chickpeas, diced tomatoes, coconut milk, curry powder, turmeric, salt, and pepper.

Bring to a simmer and cook for 20-25 minutes or until cauliflower is tender.

Garnish with fresh cilantro before serving.

Health Benefits:

Cauliflower is a low-calorie, nutrient-rich vegetable.

Chickpeas provide plant-based protein.

Cooking Time: Approximately 25 minutes

16. Greek Turkey Meatballs with Tzatziki Sauce

Ingredients:

1 pound ground turkey

1/2 cup whole wheat breadcrumbs

1/4 cup feta cheese, crumbled

1/4 cup red onion, finely chopped

2 cloves garlic, minced

1 teaspoon dried oregano

Salt and pepper to taste

Tzatziki sauce for serving

Instructions:

Preheat the oven to 375°F (190°C).

In a bowl, mix ground turkey, breadcrumbs, feta cheese, red onion, garlic, oregano, salt, and pepper.

Form the mixture into meatballs and place on a baking sheet.

Bake for 20-25 minutes or until meatballs are cooked through.

Serve with tzatziki sauce.

Health Benefits:

Ground turkey is a lean protein source.

Feta cheese adds flavor with moderate fat content.

Cooking Time: Approximately 25 minutes

17. Caprese Salad with Balsamic Glaze

Ingredients:

4 large tomatoes, sliced

1 ball fresh mozzarella, sliced

Fresh basil leaves

Balsamic glaze for drizzling

Salt and pepper to taste

Instructions:

Arrange tomato and mozzarella slices on a serving platter.

Tuck fresh basil leaves between the tomato and mozzarella slices.

Drizzle balsamic glaze over the top.

Sprinkle with salt and pepper.

Health Benefits:

Tomatoes provide vitamins and antioxidants.

Fresh mozzarella offers a creamy texture with moderate fat content.

Cooking Time: Approximately 10 minutes (no cooking required)

18. Mediterranean Quinoa Bowl

Ingredients:

1 cup cooked quinoa

1/2 cup hummus

1 cucumber, diced

1 cup cherry tomatoes, halved

1/4 cup Kalamata olives, sliced

1/4 cup feta cheese, crumbled

Fresh parsley, chopped

Lemon wedges for serving

Instructions:

In a bowl, layer cooked quinoa, hummus, diced cucumber, cherry tomatoes, olives, and feta.

Garnish with fresh parsley.

Serve with lemon wedges on the side.

Health Benefits:

Quinoa provides protein and essential nutrients.

Hummus offers plant-based protein and healthy fats.

Cooking Time: Approximately 15 minutes (assuming quinoa is pre-cooked)

19. Sweet Potato and Black Bean Chili

Ingredients:

2 sweet potatoes, peeled and diced

1 can (15 oz) black beans, drained and rinsed

1 can (14 oz) diced tomatoes

1 onion, chopped

2 cloves garlic, minced

1 tablespoon chili powder

1 teaspoon cumin

Salt and pepper to taste

Fresh cilantro for garnish

Instructions:

In a large pot, sauté onions and garlic until softened.

Add sweet potatoes, black beans, diced tomatoes, chili powder, cumin, salt, and pepper.

Bring to a boil, then reduce heat and simmer for 25-30 minutes or until sweet potatoes are tender.

Garnish with fresh cilantro before serving.

Health Benefits:

Sweet potatoes are rich in vitamins and fiber.

Black beans provide plant-based protein and fiber.

Cooking Time: Approximately 30 minutes

20. Teriyaki Salmon Bowls with Vegetables

Ingredients:

2 salmon fillets

1 cup broccoli florets

1 carrot, julienned

1 red bell pepper, sliced

1 cup snap peas

2 tablespoons low-sodium teriyaki sauce

1 tablespoon sesame seeds for garnish

Green onions, sliced, for garnish

Brown rice for serving

Instructions:

Preheat the oven to 400°F (200°C).

Place salmon fillets on a baking sheet.

Surround the salmon with broccoli, carrot, bell pepper, and snap peas.

Brush salmon and vegetables with teriyaki sauce.

Bake for 15-20 minutes or until salmon is cooked through.

Serve over brown rice and garnish with sesame seeds and sliced green onions.

Health Benefits:

Salmon provides omega-3 fatty acids.

Vegetables offer essential vitamins and minerals.

Cooking Time: Approximately 20 minutes

Certainly! Here are 20 more heart-healthy recipes suitable for an AFib-friendly diet, along with ingredients, instructions, health benefits, and estimated cooking times:

21. Chickpea and Vegetable Stir-Fry

Ingredients:

1 can (15 oz) chickpeas, drained and rinsed

2 cups broccoli florets

1 red bell pepper, sliced

1 cup snap peas

2 tablespoons low-sodium soy sauce

1 tablespoon hoisin sauce

1 tablespoon sesame oil

1 teaspoon ginger, grated

2 cloves garlic, minced

Brown rice for serving

Instructions:

In a wok or skillet, heat sesame oil over medium-high heat.

Add chickpeas, broccoli, bell pepper, snap peas, ginger, and garlic. Stir-fry until vegetables are crisp-tender.

In a small bowl, mix soy sauce and hoisin sauce. Pour over the stir-fry and toss to combine.

Serve over brown rice.

Health Benefits:

Chickpeas provide plant-based protein and fiber.

Vegetables offer essential vitamins and antioxidants.

Cooking Time: Approximately 15 minutes

22. Lemon Herb Baked Cod

Ingredients:

4 cod fillets

2 tablespoons olive oil

1 lemon, juiced and zested

2 cloves garlic, minced

1 teaspoon dried thyme

1 teaspoon dried rosemary

Salt and pepper to taste

Instructions:

Preheat the oven to 400°F (200°C).

Place cod fillets on a baking sheet.

In a small bowl, whisk together olive oil, lemon juice, lemon zest, garlic, thyme, rosemary, salt, and pepper.

Brush the mixture over the cod fillets.

Bake for 15-20 minutes or until the cod is flaky.

Health Benefits:

Cod is a lean source of protein.

Lemon and herbs add flavor without extra calories.

Cooking Time: Approximately 20 minutes

23. Mushroom and Spinach Quiche with Whole Wheat Crust

Ingredients:

1 whole wheat pie crust

1 cup mushrooms, sliced

2 cups fresh spinach, chopped

1 cup cherry tomatoes, halved

4 large eggs

1 cup skim milk

1/2 cup feta cheese, crumbled

Salt and pepper to taste

Instructions:

Preheat the oven to 375°F (190°C).

In a skillet, sauté mushrooms until softened. Add spinach and cook until wilted.

Place the whole wheat pie crust in a pie dish.

In a bowl, whisk together eggs, milk, feta, salt, and pepper.

Spread the mushroom and spinach mixture over the pie crust. Pour the egg mixture over the top.

Arrange cherry tomatoes on the surface.

Bake for 35-40 minutes or until the quiche is set.

Health Benefits:

Whole wheat crust adds fiber.

Spinach provides essential nutrients.

Cooking Time: Approximately 40 minutes

24. Vegetarian Stuffed Bell Peppers

Ingredients:

4 bell peppers, halved

1 cup cooked brown rice

1 can (15 oz) black beans, drained and rinsed

1 cup corn kernels (fresh or frozen)

1 cup salsa

1 teaspoon cumin

1 teaspoon chili powder

Shredded cheese for topping

Instructions:

Preheat the oven to 375°F (190°C).

In a bowl, mix brown rice, black beans, corn, salsa, cumin, and chili powder.

Stuff each bell pepper half with the mixture.

Top with shredded cheese.

Bake for 25-30 minutes or until peppers are tender.

Health Benefits:

Brown rice provides whole grains.

Black beans offer plant-based protein and fiber.

Cooking Time: Approximately 30 minutes

25. Cabbage and Turkey Sauté

Ingredients:

1 pound ground turkey

1 small head cabbage, thinly sliced

1 onion, chopped

2 cloves garlic, minced

1 teaspoon ground turmeric

1 teaspoon ground cumin

1/2 teaspoon paprika

Salt and pepper to taste

Instructions:

In a large skillet, cook ground turkey until browned.

Add onions and garlic, sauté until softened.

Stir in sliced cabbage, turmeric, cumin, paprika, salt, and pepper.

Sauté until cabbage is tender.

Serve as is or over quinoa.

Health Benefits:

Ground turkey is a lean protein source.

Cabbage is rich in vitamins and antioxidants.

Cooking Time: Approximately 20 minutes

26. Turkey and Vegetable Lettuce Wraps

Ingredients:

1 pound ground turkey

1 cup carrots, julienned

1 cup water chestnuts, chopped

1/4 cup hoisin sauce

2 tablespoons low-sodium soy sauce

1 tablespoon ginger, minced

Iceberg or butter lettuce leaves

Instructions:

In a skillet, cook ground turkey until browned.

Add carrots, water chestnuts, hoisin sauce, soy sauce, and ginger. Cook until vegetables are tender.

Spoon the turkey mixture into lettuce leaves to create wraps.

Serve immediately.

Health Benefits:

Ground turkey is a lean protein source.

Lettuce wraps offer a low-carb alternative to traditional wraps.

Cooking Time: Approximately 15 minutes

27. Pesto Zoodles with Cherry Tomatoes

Ingredients:

4 zucchinis, spiralized into zoodles

1 cup cherry tomatoes, halved

1/4 cup pesto sauce

2 tablespoons pine nuts, toasted

Parmesan cheese for garnish (optional)

Instructions:

In a large pan, sauté zoodles until slightly softened.

Add cherry tomatoes and cook until heated through.

Stir in pesto sauce and toss until zoodles are well-coated.

Top with toasted pine nuts and Parmesan cheese if desired.

Health Benefits:

Zucchini provides a low-calorie, nutrient-rich base.

Pesto sauce adds flavor without excessive calories.

Cooking Time: Approximately 10 minutes

28. Eggplant and Lentil Moussaka

Ingredients:

2 eggplants, sliced

1 cup cooked green or brown lentils

1 onion, finely chopped

3 cloves garlic, minced

1 can (14 oz) diced tomatoes

1 teaspoon dried oregano

1 teaspoon ground cinnamon

1/2 cup plain Greek yogurt

2 tablespoons grated Parmesan cheese

Instructions:

Preheat the oven to 375°F (190°C).

Grill or roast eggplant slices until tender.

In a skillet, sauté onions and garlic until softened.

Add cooked lentils, diced tomatoes, oregano, and cinnamon. Simmer until heated through.

In a baking dish, layer grilled eggplant and lentil mixture.

Top with Greek yogurt and Parmesan cheese.

Bake for 25-30 minutes or until bubbly and golden.

Health Benefits:

Eggplant is low in calories and rich in antioxidants.

Lentils provide plant-based protein and fiber.

Cooking Time: Approximately 30 minutes

29. Lemon Garlic Shrimp with Quinoa

Ingredients:

1 cup quinoa, cooked

1 pound shrimp, peeled and deveined

2 tablespoons olive oil

3 cloves garlic, minced

Zest and juice of 1 lemon

1 teaspoon dried thyme

Fresh parsley for garnish

Salt and pepper to taste

Instructions:

In a skillet, heat olive oil over medium-high heat.

Add shrimp and cook until pink.

Stir in garlic, lemon zest, lemon juice, dried thyme, salt, and pepper.

Serve over cooked quinoa.

Garnish with fresh parsley.

Health Benefits:

Shrimp provides lean protein.

Quinoa offers whole grains and essential nutrients.

Cooking Time: Approximately 15 minutes

30. Stuffed Acorn Squash with Wild Rice and Cranberries

Ingredients:

2 acorn squashes, halved and seeds removed

1 cup wild rice, cooked

1/2 cup dried cranberries

1/4 cup pecans, chopped

2 tablespoons maple syrup

1 tablespoon olive oil

Fresh thyme for garnish

Salt and pepper to taste

Instructions:

Preheat the oven to 400°F (200°C).

Place acorn squash halves on a baking sheet.

In a bowl, mix cooked wild rice, dried cranberries, chopped pecans, maple syrup, olive oil, salt, and pepper.

Stuff each acorn squash half with the rice mixture.

Bake for 30-35 minutes or until squash is tender.

Garnish with fresh thyme before serving.

Health Benefits:

Wild rice provides whole grains.

Cranberries add antioxidants and natural sweetness.

Cooking Time: Approximately 35 minutes

CONCLUSION

Incorporating heart-healthy recipes into your diet not only supports overall cardiovascular well-being but also provides a delicious and diverse array of flavors to enjoy. These recipes, carefully curated with ingredients known for their cardiovascular benefits, offer a mix of lean proteins, whole grains, fruits, vegetables, and essential nutrients. Whether you're looking for seafood dishes rich in omega-3 fatty acids, plant-based options filled with fiber, or flavorful combinations that tantalize your taste buds, these recipes cater to various dietary preferences.

Remember, maintaining a heart-healthy lifestyle involves more than just individual meals; it's about embracing a balanced and sustainable approach to nutrition. Adjust these recipes to suit your taste, dietary requirements, and portion preferences. Additionally, consult with healthcare professionals or a nutritionist to personalize your dietary plan based on your unique health needs.